The Best Mediterranean Meals & Desserts

50 Mouth-Watering Sweet & Savory Mediterranean Recipes

Carmen Berlanti

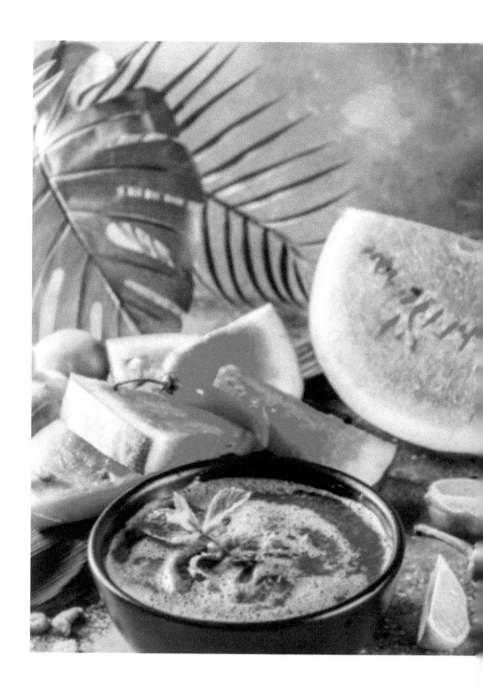

Table of Contents

Eggs over Kale Hash

Difficulty Level: 2/5

Preparation time: 10 minutes

Cooking time: 20 minutes

Servings: 4

Ingredients:

4 large eggs

1 bunch chopped kale

Dash of ground nutmeg

2 sweet potatoes, cubed

1 14.5-ounce can of chicken broth

Directions:

In a large non-stick skillet, bring the chicken broth to a simmer. Add the sweet potatoes and season slightly with salt and pepper.

Add a dash of nutmeg to improve the flavor.

Cook until the sweet potatoes become soft, around 10 minutes. Add kale and season with salt and pepper. Continue cooking for four minutes or until kale has wilted. Set aside.

Using the same skillet, heat 1 tablespoon of olive oil over medium high heat.

Cook the eggs sunny side up until the whites become opaque and the yolks have set. Top the kale hash with the eggs. Serve immediately.

Nutrition:

Calories per serving: 158;

Protein: 9.8g;

Carbohydrates 18.5g;

Fat: 5.6g

Italian Scrambled Eggs

Difficulty Level: 2/5

Preparation time: 5 minutes

Cooking Time: 7 minutes

Servings: 1

Ingredients:

1 teaspoon balsamic vinegar

2 large eggs

¼ teaspoon rosemary, minced

½ cup cherry tomatoes

1 ½ cup kale, chopped

½ teaspoon olive oil

Directions:

Melt the olive oil in a skillet over medium high heat.

Sauté the kale and add rosemary and salt to taste. Add three tablespoons of water to prevent the kale from burning at the bottom of the pan. Cook for three to four minutes.

Add the tomatoes and stir.

Push the vegetables on one side of the skillet and add the eggs. Season with salt and pepper to taste.

Scramble the eggs then fold in the tomatoes and kales.

Nutrition:

Calories per serving: 230;

Protein: 16.4g;

Carbs: 15.0g;

Fat: 12.4g

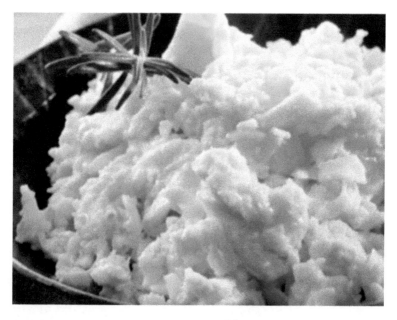

Scrambled Eggs with Feta 'n Mushrooms

Difficulty Level: 2/5

Preparation time: 5 minutes

Cooking time: 6 minutes

Servings: 1

Ingredients:

Pepper to taste

2 tbsp feta cheese

1 whole egg

2 egg whites

1 cup fresh spinach, chopped

½ cup fresh mushrooms, sliced

Cooking spray

Directions:

On medium high fire, place a nonstick fry pan and grease with cooking spray.

Once hot, add spinach and mushrooms.

Sauté until spinach is wilted, around 2-3 minutes.

Meanwhile, in a bowl whisk well egg, egg whites, and cheese. Season with pepper.

Pour egg mixture into pan and scramble until eggs are cooked through, around 3-4 minutes.

Serve and enjoy with a piece of toast or brown rice.

Nutrition:

Calories per serving: 211;

Protein: 18.6g;

Carbs: 7.4g;

Fat: 11.9g

Black Bean Hummus

Difficulty Level: 2/5

Preparation time: 5 min

Cooking time: -min

Servings: 2

Ingredients:

2 (15.5 ounce) cans black beans

2 cups low-fat cottage cheese

3 tablespoons almond butter

1 garlic clove, sliced

2 tablespoons extra-virgin olive oil

3 tablespoons red wine vinegar

3/4 teaspoon sea salt

1/2 teaspoon ground cumin

1 teaspoon ground coriander

1/4 cup fresh parsley

2 tablespoons orange zest

Freshly ground black pepper to taste

10-12 stalks of celery, cut into thirds

Directions:

Mix all the ingredients in a food processor, except celery, and puree till smooth. If necessary, scrap down the sides.

Move to a bowl and serve with celery. *Enjoy!*

Nutrition: (Per serving)

Calories:218kcal;

Fat:7.5g;

Saturated fat:1.5g;

Cholesterol:10mg;

Carbohydrate:20g;

Sugar:4.5g;

Fiber:5.5g;

Protein:16g

Portobello Mushroom Delight

Difficulty Level: 2/5

Preparation time: 5 min

Cooking time: 15 min

Servings: 2

Ingredients:

2 Portobello mushroom caps (around 3 ounces each)

2 tablespoons soft goat cheese

2 tablespoons sundried tomatoes

2 large eggs

extra-virgin (organic) olive oil spray

Salt and pepper to taste

Basil for garnish

Directions:

Preheat the oven to 400 degrees Fahrenheit.

From the mushroom caps remove the stems and with a spoon scrape out the gills.

Use cooking spray to spray both sides of the mushroom and set them onto the baking sheet.

Place into each mushroom 1 tablespoon of goat cheese, where the gills used to be.

Finely chop sun-dried tomatoes and sprinkle into each mushroom cap 1 tablespoon of them.

Into each mushroom cap crack an egg, striving to get the yolk to sit in the cavity where the steam was, so it doesn't move around.

Transfer the baking sheet to the oven and bake for 15 minutes.

Once the eggs are done to your liking, transfer them from the oven and season with salt and pepper.

Top with sliced basil and serve. *Enjoy!*

Tip: Make this into a meal by tossing arugula, baby kale, or other lettuce greens in lemon juice, olive oil, salt and pepper and having as a side salad.

Nutrition: (Per serving)

Calories:122kcal;

Fat:8.5g;

Saturated fat:3g;

Cholesterol:223mg;

Carbohydrate:2g;

Sugar:1g;

Fiber:0.5g;

Protein:8.5g

Tuna Salad On Crackers

Difficulty Level: 1/5

Preparation time: 10 min

Cooking time: - min

Servings: 4

Ingredients:

1 (7 ounce) can Albacore Tuna in brine water

2 tablespoons celery, finely chopped

3 tablespoons Canola Oil Mayonnaise

1/2 teaspoon lemon pepper

11/2 tablespoons red onion, finely chopped

1/4 teaspoon dried dill weed

16 Ritz Crackers

2 green leaf lettuce leaves, torn

Fresh dill, for garnish (optional)

Directions:

In a mixing bowl place tuna and mash up to desired size pieces. Add in celery, mayonnaise, lemon pepper, onion, and dill weed. Mix well to combine.

On top of each cracker place a piece of torn lettuce and top that with 1 tablespoon of tuna salad. Decorate with a piece of fresh dill weed, if desired and serve. *Enjoy!*

Nutrition (4 crackers)

Calories:165kcal;

Fat:7g;

Saturated fat:1g;

Cholesterol:19mg;

Carbohydrate:9g;

Sugar:1g;

Fiber:1g;

Protein:13g

Fresh Fruit Crumble Muesli

Difficulty Level: 1/5

Preparation Time: *20 minutes*

Cooking Time: *0 minutes*

Servings: *4*

Ingredients:

1 cup gluten-free rolled oats

¼ cup chopped pecans

¼ cup almonds

4 pitted Medjool dates

1 teaspoon vanilla extract

¼ teaspoon ground cinnamon

1 cup sliced fresh strawberries

1 nectarine, pitted and chopped

2 kiwis, peeled and chopped

½ cup blueberries

1 cup low-fat plain Greek yogurt

Directions:

In a food processor, combine the oats, pecans, almonds, dates, vanilla, and cinnamon and pulse until the mixture resembles coarse crumbs.

In a medium bowl, stir together the strawberries, nectarine, kiwis, and blueberries until well mixed. Divide the fruit and yogurt between bowls and top each bowl with the oat mixture. Serve.

Nutrition:

Calories: 258

Total fat: 6g

Saturated fat: 0g

Carbohydrates: 45g

Sugar: 28g

Fiber: 7g

Protein: 11g

Crispy Squid with Capers

Difficulty Level: 2/5

Preparation Time: 5 minutes

Cooking time: 20 minutes

Servings: 3

Ingredients:

1 garlic clove, crushed

2½ tablespoons mayonnaise

Olive oil, for frying

3.5 oz. whole wheat flour

5 oz. baby squid, cleaned and sliced into thick rings

1 tablespoon caper, drained and finely chopped

Lemon wedges, to serve

Directions:

Combine together squid, capers and whole wheat flour in a bowl.

Heat oil in a skillet and deep fry capers and squids until golden.

Dish out the capers and squid in a plate.

Serve with mayonnaise, garlic and lemon wedges.

Nutrition:

Calories 213

Total Fat 5.1 g

Saturated Fat 0.8 g

Cholesterol 113 mg

Total Carbs 29.9 g

Dietary Fiber 1 g

Sugar 0.9 g

Protein 11 g

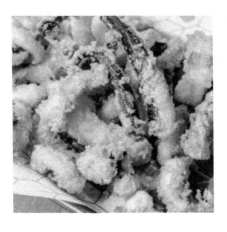

Garlic Bread Pizzas

Difficulty Level: 2/5

Preparation Time: 10 minutes

Cooking time: 15 minutes

Servings: 8

Ingredients:

For the dough

2 pounds strong whole wheat flour, plus extra for rolling

4 tablespoons olive oil

2 sachets fast-action yeast

2 teaspoons salt

For the topping

½ cup almond butter, softened

2 teaspoons balsamic vinegar

2 tablespoons extra-virgin olive oil

4 garlic cloves, crushed

3 cups mozzarella, drained

½ cup basil leaves, roughly chopped

8 tomatoes, roughly chopped

Directions:

Preheat the oven to 330 degrees F and grease 4 baking sheets.

Knead together all the ingredients for the dough in a bowl and roll out into 16 equal pieces.

Mix together garlic and butter in a bowl and pour over the dough.

Organize these pieces into the baking sheets and top with mozzarella cheese.

Transfer into the oven and bake for about 15 minutes.

Top with rest of the ingredients and immediately serve.

Nutrition:

Calories 629

Total Fat 21.8 g

Saturated Fat 9.6 g

Cholesterol 36 mg

Total Carbs 92.2 g

Dietary Fiber 4.6 g

Sugar 3.6 g

Protein 16 g

Falafel

Difficulty Level: 2/5

Preparation Time: 15 minutes

Cooking time: 4 minutes

Servings: 6

Ingredients:

1 cup chickpeas, cooked

1 onion, finely chopped

2 tablespoons flour

1 tablespoon chopped parsley

1 teaspoon ground coriander

2 tablespoons olive oil

1 teaspoon salt

Directions:

Blend the cooked chickpeas, chopped onion, and parsley.

When the mixture is smooth, add the flour and ground coriander.

Blend the mixture for 20 seconds more.

Transfer the mixture to bowl.

Make small balls from the chickpea mixture and press them gently into a flat disc.

Pour the olive oil into the pressure pot bowl.

Add the falafel and use the saute mode to cook the falafel for 2 minutes on each side.

Cool the cooked falafel slightly and serve!

Nutrition:

Calories 178,

Fat 6.7,

Fiber 6.3,

Carbs 23.9,

Protein 6.9

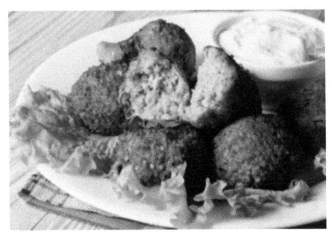

Chicken Sandwich

Difficulty Level: 2/5

 Preparation Time: 10 minutes

Cooking time: 15 minutes

Servings: 4

Ingredients:

7 oz. chicken fillets

1 tablespoon olive oil

1 teaspoon salts

½ teaspoon ground black pepper

4 oz. French bread, sliced

1 tomato, sliced

1 cup water

2 oz. lettuce

Directions:

Cut the chicken fillet into strips.

Sprinkle the chicken with the salt and ground black pepper.

Add the olive oil and stir the meat well.

Pour the water into the pressure pot.

Place the trivet in the pressure pot and put the chicken strips on the trivet.

Cook the chicken using steam mode for 15 minutes.

Do a natural pressure release.

Meanwhile, place the lettuce and sliced tomato on the bread slices.

Add the cooked chicken strips to make the sandwiches.

Enjoy!

Nutrition:

Calories 212,

Fat 7.8,

Fiber 1,

Carbs 17.2,

Protein 17.9

Mediterranean Creamy Deviled Eggs

Difficulty Level: 2/5

Preparation Time: 10 minutes

Cooking time: 2 minutes

Servings: 4

Ingredients:

2 eggs

1 cup water

1 tablespoon cream

1 teaspoon mayo

½ teaspoon ground black pepper

1 teaspoon oregano

1 teaspoon cilantro

Directions:

Pour the water into the pressure pot.

Add the eggs and close the lid.

Cook the eggs on High pressure for 2 minutes.

Do a natural pressure release.

Cool the eggs in the ice water.

Peel the eggs.

Cut the eggs into halves and remove the egg yolks.

Put the egg yolks, mayo, ground black pepper, oregano, cilantro, and cream in a blender.

Blend the mixture well.

Fill the egg whites with the egg yolk mixture.

Enjoy!

Nutrition:

Calories 53,

Fat 4.2,

Fiber 0.2,

Carbs 1.2,

Protein 2.9

Fish Scones

Difficulty Level: 2/5

Preparation Time: 15 minutes

Cooking time: 10 minutes

Servings: 8

Ingredients:

8 oz. puff pastry

7 oz. tuna, canned

1 egg, whisked

1 teaspoon salt

1 teaspoon ground coriander

½ teaspoon ground black pepper

1 tablespoon olive oil

1 teaspoon dried dill

Directions:

Roll out the puff pastry.

Combine the whisked egg, canned tuna, salt, ground coriander, ground black pepper, and dried dill.

Stir the mixture well.

Cut the puff pastry into medium squares.

Place a small amount of the tuna mixture in each puff pastry square.

Secure the edges of the puff pastry in the shape of the scones.

Sprinkle the scones with the olive oil.

Place the scones in a baking pan and place the pan in the pressure pot bowl.

Cook the fish scones for 10 minutes on High pressure.

Do a natural pressure release.

Serve the cooked scones and enjoy!

Nutrition Value:

Calories 226,

Fat 15.1,

Fiber 0.5,

Carbs 13,

Protein 9.4

Green Beans with Yogurt Drizzle

Difficulty Level: 2/5

Preparation time: 10 minutes

Cooking time: 5 minutes

Servings: 4

Ingredients:

1 pound of green beans (thin, trimmed)

3 tablespoons extra-virgin olive oil (divided)

1 red bell pepper (chopped)

1/2 cup Greek yogurt

1/4 cup grated Parmesan cheese

2 lemon juice teaspoons

1/2 teaspoon anchovy paste

1 clove garlic (chopped)

black olives (very small, for garnish)

fresh parsley (for garnish)

Directions:

Steam or cook green beans in boiling water to desired softness. Drain. Heat 1 tablespoon oil in a skillet and cook 10-inch pepper over medium heat, stirring occasionally for 4 minutes or until softened.

Add green beans and toss to coat. Combine remaining ingredients except olives in a microwave-safe bowl and cook at HIGH temp. for 30 seconds, stirring once, until warm.

Arrange green beans on a serving platter. Top with red peppers and olives. Serve sauce over vegetables. Garnish with fresh parsley leaves.

Nutrition: (Per serving)
190 Calories;

0.14g fat;

0.12g carbs;

0.6g protein;

Roast Vegetables with Tomatoes, Feta and Basil

Difficulty Level: 2/5

Preparation time: 15 minutes

Cooking time: 15 minutes

Servings: 4

Ingredients:

zucchini (thinly sliced, about 200 g)

olive oil

salt

pepper

2 cloves

eggplant (cut into small cubes, approximately 200 g)

bell pepper (medium size, color of your choice, cut into small cubes, 1)

cherry tomatoes (cut in half, 8)

feta cheese (broken into pieces, approximately 100 g / 3 1/2 oz)

10 fresh basil leaves

Directions:

Heat a slash or olive oil in a large pan and sauté the zucchini on medium-high heat until golden brown with a little bite. Season with salt and pepper to taste, transfer to a plate and set aside.

Put the pan back on the heat, pour in a splash of olive oil, stir in the garlic and let it turn golden (not brown!) For about 1 minute. Add the eggplant and bell pepper, season with salt and pepper and sauté until golden and soft. Take the pan off the heat, mix in the zucchini and tomatoes and season to taste. Stir in the feta and basil and serve immediately, or as a warm salad, with fresh ciabatta bread.

Nutrition: (Per serving)
90 Calories;

0.7g fat;

0.6g carbs;

0.2g protein;

Roasted Broccoli & Tomatoes

Difficulty Level: 2/5

Preparation time: 5 minutes

Cooking time: 20 minutes

Servings: 4

Ingredients:

12 ounces of broccoli (crowns, trimmed and cut into bite-size florets, about 4 cups)

1 cup grape tomatoes

1 tablespoon extra-virgin olive oil

2 cloves of garlic

1/4 teaspoon salt

1/2 teaspoon grated lemon zest (freshly)

1 tablespoon lemon juice

10 pitted black olives (sliced)

1 teaspoon of dried oregano

2 teaspoons capers (rinsed, optional)

Directions:

Preheat oven to 450 ° F.

Throw broccoli, tomatoes, oil, garlic and salt in a large bowl until evenly covered. Spread in an even layer on a baking sheet. Bake until the broccoli starts to brown, 10 to 13 minutes.

Meanwhile, mix lemon zest and juice, olives, oregano and capers (if used) in a large bowl. Add the roasted vegetables; stir to combine. Serve hot.

Nutrition: (Per serving)

70 Calories;

0.35g fat;

0.9g carbs;

0.3g protein

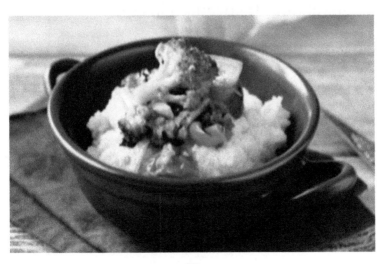

Grilled Zucchini with Tomato and Feta

Difficulty Level: 2/5

Preparation time: 5 minutes

Cooking time: 12 minutes

Servings: 6

Ingredients:

3 zucchini (or zucchini and yellow squash, tops removed, cut in half lengthwise)

freshly ground pepper (bars)

1/2 teaspoon of garlic powder

extra virgin olive oil

1/2 lemon (about 1 tbsp lemon juice)

1 whole lemon

1/2 cup of crumbled feta cheese

3 pearl tomatoes (chopped, drained in a colander)

1 green onion (both white and green, finely chopped)

Directions:

If cooking on gas grill, lightly oil the grate and preheat grill to medium-low. (OR, heat and cast iron skillet or indoor griddle over medium heat.)

Brush zucchini generously with extra virgin olive oil on both sides. Season zucchini (particularly flesh side) with salt, freshly ground pepper, and oregano

Place zucchini, flesh-side down, on the preheated grill (or indoor griddle). Grill for 3 to 5 minutes until soft and nicely charred, then turn on back side and grill for another 3 to 5 minutes until this side is also tender and gains some color. (If using an indoor skillet or griddle, you may need to adjust heat to medium-high.)

Remove zucchini from heat and let's cool enough to handle.

To create zucchini boats, use a small spoon to scoop out the flesh into a small bowl (do not discard.) Squeeze all liquid out of zucchini flesh (you might use a linen kitchen towel or paper towel to do this.)

Now add zucchini flesh to a mixing bowl. Add the remaining ingredients (cherry tomatoes, green onions, feta, mint, parsley, lemon zest, and small splash or lemon juice). Sprinkle a little more oregano, if you like, and add a drizzle or extra virgin olive oil. Mix everything together to make the filling.

Spoon the filling mixture into the prepared zucchini boats and arrange on a serving platter. Enjoy!

Nutrition: (Per serving)

90 Calories;

0.6g fat;

0.7g carbs;

0.3g protein;

0mg of cholesterol;

150mg sodium

Taziki's Mediterranean Cafés Basmati Rice

Difficulty Level: 2/5

Preparation time: 10 minutes

Cooking time: 20 minutes

Servings: 4

Ingredients:

2 cups basmati rice (long grain Indian Basmati rice)

3 cups of water

4 ounces of unsalted butter (melted)

1 teaspoon of salt

1 teaspoon pepper

4 lemon juice (lemons)

1/2 cup parsley (fresh chopped)

Directions:

Put water and rice in an 8-liter pan with a lid.

Bring the rice to the boil quickly while it is covered.

When the water boils, set the temperature low.

Bake for 12 to 15 minutes until the rice is fluffy.

Remove the pan from the burner and let the rice stand for 2 to 5 minutes.

Pour cooked rice into a medium-sized mixing bowl.

Add melted butter, salt, pepper, lemon juice and parsley.

Stir until it has cooled completely.

Nutrition: (Per serving)

560 Calories;

0.24g fat;

0.79g carbs;

0.7g protein

Roasted Broccoli & Tomatoes

Difficulty Level: 2/5

Preparation time: 5 minutes

Cooking time: 20 minutes

Servings: 4

Ingredients:

12 ounces of broccoli (crowns, trimmed and cut into bite-size florets, about 4 cups)

1 cup grape tomatoes

1 tablespoon extra-virgin olive oil

2 cloves of garlic (minced)

1/4 teaspoon salt

1/2 teaspoon grated lemon zest (freshly)

1 tablespoon lemon juice

10 pitted black olives (sliced)

1 teaspoon of dried oregano

2 teaspoons capers (rinsed, optional)

Directions:

Preheat oven to 450 ° F. Toss broccoli, tomatoes, oil, garlic and salt in a large bowl until evenly coated. Spread in an even layer on a baking sheet. Bake until the broccoli starts to brown, 10 to 13 minutes.

Meanwhile, combine lemon zest and juice, olives, oregano and capers (if using) in a large bowl. Add the roasted vegetables; stir to combine. Serve hot.

Nutrition: (Per serving)

70 Calories;

0.35g fat;

0.9g carbs;

0.3g protein;

Green Beans Mediterranean Style

Difficulty Level: 2/5

Preparation time: 5 minutes

Cooking time: 10 minutes

Servings: 6

Ingredients:

12 ounces of haricot verts (Fresh, French Green Beans, See Note 1)

1 1/2 cups cherry tomatoes

1/3 cup pitted kalamata olives (Small)

2 cups bread cubes (1/2 ", See Note 2)

1/2 oregano teaspoon

1/2 teaspoon of salt

4 tablespoons extra virgin olive oil (divided)

1/4 teaspoon Dijon mustard

1 tablespoon balsamic vinegar (White)

1 ounce of feta cheese

1 pinch red pepper flake

Directions:

Preheat oven to 375 ºF (Conventional), or 350 ºF for Convection (fan).

In a large bowl, place the green beans, tomatoes, olives and bread cubes. Drizzle with 3 T olive oil, the oregano, and 1/2 t salt. Mix until all pieces are coated.

Spread onto large Sheet Pan.

Place in oven for 15-20 minutes, until croutons are crispy, and beans are tender. In my oven, this took about 18 minutes

Make the dressing. In a small container with a member, mix the Dijon mustard, balsamic vinegar and the remaining tablespoon of olive oil. Add a pinch of salt and a few changes to freshly ground pepper. Sprinkle with the green beans. Place in a serving dish.

Crumble and sprinkle the feta cheese and a pinch of red pepper flake (if desired) over the top and serve while it is hot.

Nutrition: (Per serving)

160 Calories;

0.11g fat;

0.13g carbs;

0.3g protein;

Italian-style Broccoli

Difficulty Level: 2/5

Preparation time: 5 minutes

Cooking time: 25 minutes

Servings: 4

Ingredients:

3 cloves of garlic (diced)

1/2 yellow onion (diced)

3 tablespoons olive oil

1 pound broccoli florets (steamed, fresh or frozen)

1/4 cup black olives (finely chopped)

3/4 teaspoon of salt

Directions:

About medium heat, sauté the onion and garlic in the oil for 2-3 minutes until the onions start to turn color.

Add in the broccoli and lower the heat. Toss the pan to make sure the broccoli soaks up the oil.

Also add in the olives and distribute throughout the dish. Serve hot.

Nutrition: (Per serving)

150 Calories;

0.11g fat;

0.10g carbs;

0.4g protein;

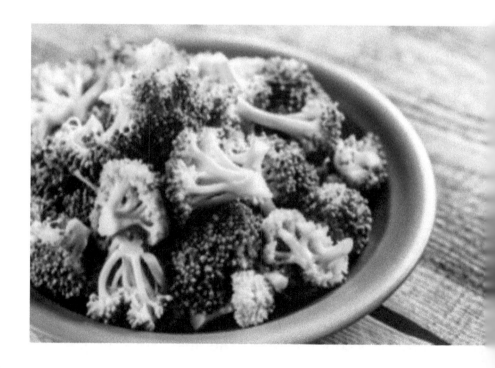

Zucchini Mediterranean

Difficulty Level: 2/5

Preparation time: 5 minutes

Cooking time: 25 minutes

Servings: 4

Ingredients:

4 zucchini

2 tablespoons olive oil

2 tablespoons of vinegar

1 garlic (mashed)

1/2 teaspoon basil

1/2 oregano teaspoon

salt (to taste)

pepper (to taste)

Directions:

Wash, trim, and slice zucchini

Saute in oil until slightly soft.

Drizzle vinegar about zucchini while cooking.

Add garlic, basil, oregano, salt, and pepper.

Toss to coat well.

Serve hot or cold.

Nutrition: (Per serving)

100 Calories;

0.7g fat;

0.8g carbs;

0.2g protein

Greek Couscous

Difficulty Level: 2/5

Preparation time: 5 minutes

Cooking time: 20 minutes

Servings: 4

Ingredients:

1 cup of couscous

1 cup of water

2/3 cup peppers (diced, sweet, bell ... whatever suits your fancy)

1/2 cup sun-dried tomatoes (diced)

2/3 cup kalamata olives (chopped)

3 tablespoons juices (oils from tomatoes and olives)

4 ounces of crumbled feta cheese

parsley (generous sprinkle or, I used dried, but you can use fresh if you have it)

Directions:

Prepare couscous as indicated on the package. (Mine says to boil the water, add couscous, stir quickly and remove from the heat; let stand for 5 minutes). I have skipped both butter and salt.

Mix the peppers, tomatoes and olives well in a large bowl.

Add couscous and stir, breaking up the large pieces.

Add the juices and / or oils from the tomatoes and olive to the couscous as needed to keep dish moist, but not wet. Couscous will absorb liquid quickly, so be generous and work fast.

Once the couscous and vegetables are mixed well, add feta and stir to combine.

Sprinkle parsley just before serving. Enjoy!

Nutrition: (Per serving)

330 Calories;

0.1g fat;

0.52g carbs;

0.13g protein;

Mushroom Couscous

Difficulty Level: 2/5

Preparation time: 5 minutes

Cooking time: *30 minutes*

Servings: 4

Ingredients:

1/2 cup couscous (uncooked)

1 cup of water

1 tablespoon butter

7 mushrooms (sliced)

2 carrots (sliced & cooked)

2 tablespoons chive (chopped)

1 teaspoon garlic powder

1 1/2 herb teaspoons (Italian, blend)

1 tablespoon lemon juice

salt / pepper

Directions:

Add couscous and water in a medium saucepan. Bake for 5 - 10 minutes over medium heat until the couscous is cooked.

Melt butter in a frying pan. Add sliced mushrooms and cook for 5 minutes. Add carrots, cooked couscous, chopped chives, garlic powder, Italian spice mix and lemon juice. Bake for about 5 - 10 minutes. Season with salt and pepper.

Nutrition: (Per serving)

150 Calories;

0.35g fat;

0.25g carbs;

0.5g protein

Parmesan Mashed Potatoes with Olive Oil, Garlic, & Parsley

Difficulty Level: 2/5

Preparation time: 5 minutes

Cooking time: *30 minutes*

Servings: *4*

Ingredients:

5 pounds red skinned potatoes (chopped into 2 inch pieces)

2 heads roasted garlic

4 tablespoons garlic powder

3 cups heavy cream

1/2 pound Parmesan cheese

1/4 cup fresh parsley (chopped)

1/4 cup olive oil (Pompeian, I love the Mediterranean blend!)

pepper

salt

olive oil (additional, to drizzle & fresh chopped parsley to garnish, optional)

Directions:

Boil the potatoes in enough water to cover until fork tender. Drain. Place the potatoes back into the pot on medium, and mash best you can with a potato masher to release the steam. Pour in the heavy cream, & finish mashing the potatoes. Stir the mixture to combine. Stir in the Parmesan cheese, garlic, & fresh chopped parsley. Drizzle in the olive oil, a little at a time - stirring after each drizzle, until all the olive oil is combined. Season with salt & pepper to taste.

Scoop into your serving vessel; drizzle with olive oil and sprinkle on chopped parsley to garnish if desired

Nutrition: (Per serving)

1570 Calories;

0.113g fat;

0.109g carbs;

0.38g protein;

Greek Cauliflower Rice with Feta and Olives

Difficulty Level: 2/5

Preparation time: 5 minutes

Cooking time: *30 minutes*

Servings: 4

Ingredients:

1 shallot (large, diced)

1 tablespoon coconut oil

1 pound cauliflower (aged or shredded in food processor, you can buy it pre-shredded at Trader Joe's in the products section)

1 cup of crumbled feta cheese

1/2 cup sliced black olives (kalamata is great, but every black olive does with it)

1/3 cup parsley (finely chopped, plus more for garnish)

salt

pepper

Directions:

Heat coconut oil in a frying pan over medium heat. When the oil sparkles, add the diced shallot. Sauté until transparent.

Put the cauliflower rice in the pan. Cook for 10-15 minutes, stirring occasionally. Brown the cauliflower a little and then remove from the heat. Stir in the parsley, olives and feta and season with salt and pepper. Garnish with extra parsley if desired. Serve hot.

Nutrition: (Per serving)

200 Calories;

0.13g fat;

0.15g carbs;

0.9g protein

Brussels Sprouts

Difficulty Level: 2/5

Preparation time: 5 minutes

Cooking time: *15 minutes*

Servings: *5*

Ingredients:

1 pound brussels sprouts (quartered)

1 tablespoon olive oil

1/2 oregano teaspoon

1 teaspoon crushed garlic

1/2 teaspoon of salt

1/4 teaspoon pepper

20 kalamata olives (pitted and halved)

8 sun dried tomatoes (sliced)

1/2 cup of feta cheese

1/2 cup sliced almonds (toasted)

Directions:

Cook Brussels in the microwave for 4 minutes.

Meanwhile, heat the olive oil and garlic in a large frying pan. Cook for a minute or two.

Add tomatoes, Brussels, olives, oregano, salt and pepper.

Bake for a few minutes.

In the meantime, roast for a few minutes in a dry frying pan. Be careful not to burn them.

When almonds are a little roasted. Remove everything from the stove.

Add the feta cheese and sprinkle the almonds on top and serve.

Nutrition: (Per serving)

180 Calories;

0.1g fat;

0.14g carbs;

0.8g protein

Garlic Scapes Sautéed with Olive Oil, Sea Salt & Freshly Ground Pepper

Difficulty Level: 2/5

Preparation time: 5 minutes

Cooking time: *25 minutes*

Servings: *2*

Ingredients:

1 bunch of garlic scapes (about 12 to 14 votes)

1 olive oil teaspoon

sea salt (to taste, I use Mediterranean sea salt)

freshly ground black pepper (to taste)

Directions:

Rinse garlic scapes under cold water in a colander. Cut off the hard lower part of the vote. Pat dry.

Add olive to a flat wide pan over medium high heat, heat for about a minute. Add the garlic scapes, sprinkle with salt and freshly ground pepper. Sauté for about a minute, flip the scapes over and fry on the other side.

Add about a teaspoon of water, cover the pan with a fitted member and let it steam for a few minutes until tender. Lift the member and check for done-ness. If the scapes are getting too dry but are not tender yet, add another spoon of water, cover and steam.

When the stems are tender (check with a fork), uncover and fry for another minute. Scapes should be lightly charred, they're tastier that way. Remove from heat and serve immediately.

Nutrition: (Per serving)

Calories: 301;

Protein: 17g;

Total Carbohydrates: 29g;

Sugars: 2g;

Fiber: 17g;

Total Fat: 14g;

Saturated Fat: 2g;

Watermelon Gazpacho

Difficulty Level: 2/5

Preparation time: 10 minutes

Cooking time: None

Servings: 6

Ingredients:

salt

1 seedless cucumber, chopped

1 tsp minced garlic

1 tbsp chopped fresh basil

2 celery stalks, chopped

2 ripe tomatoes, chopped

2 tbsp rice vinegar

2 tbsp chopped fresh cilantro

3 tbsp fresh lime juice

8 cups chopped seedless watermelon

Directions:

Begin with setting aside a single cup of chopped watermelon. Using a food processor place the rest of the food and begin processing.

Begin adding the celery, garlic, tomatoes, and cucumber. Continue processing until the resulting mixture is chopped well but not fully pureed.

Place the mixture into a container and begin mixing with the vinegar, herbs, salt, and lime juice.

Add the watermelon into the mixture and continue to mix. Refrigerate for a minimum of two hours and serve chilled.

Nutrition:

Calories: 132

Carbohydrates: 24 g

Fats: 5 g

Proteins: 9 g

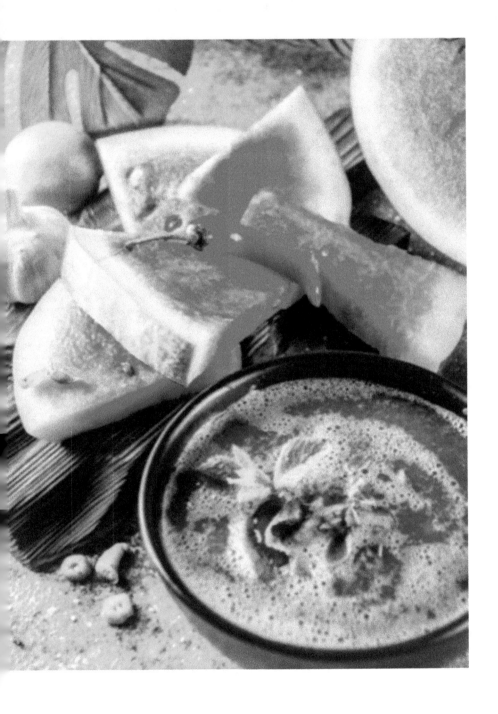

Herb-Tossed Olives

Difficulty Level: 2/5

Preparation time: 10 minutes

Cooking time: None

Servings: 4

Ingredients:

⅛ tsp dried oregano

⅛ tsp dried thyme

⅛ tsp dried basil

black pepper to taste

1 garlic clove, crushed

2 tsp extra-virgin olive oil

3 cups assorted pitted olives

Procedure:

Put the olives in a medium-sized container and add in the olive oil.

Add the garlic, herbs, and season as well as the pepper. Once added toss the entire mix.

If not going to be served immediately, ensure to refrigerate until the food is ready to be served.

Nutrition:

Calories: 281

Carbohydrates: 30 g

Fats: 4 g

Proteins: 8 g

Cucumber Mozzarella Skewers

Difficulty Level: 2/5

Preparation time: 10 minutes

Cooking time: None

Servings: 4

Ingredients:

one 8-ounce ball fresh mozzarella, thinly sliced

salt and pepper to taste

1 bunch fresh basil

1 tbsp balsamic vinegar

2 seedless cucumbers, sliced ¼ inch thick

2 tbsp extra-virgin olive oil

Directions:

Place the piece of cucumber on a plate. Arrange the cucumbers so that each one is on top of the preceding slice.

Add in the arrangement the basil leaf and mozzarella.

Sandwich the mozzarella and basil with another piece of cucumber slice and secure by skewering a piece of toothpick.

Mix the balsamic vinegar and the olive oil together, add pepper and salt to the mix.

Pour the mixture over the skewers and serve.

Nutrition:

Calories: 88

Carbohydrates: 29 g

Fats: 7 g

Proteins: 8 g

Tomato and Almond Pesto

Difficulty Level: 2/5

Preparation time: 15 minutes

Cooking time: None

Servings: 4 cups

Ingredients:

¾ Cup slivered almonds

one 28-oz. can diced tomatoes, drained

one 14-oz. can tomatoes, fire-roasted, drained

¾ cup of extra-virgin olive oil

½ cup grated parmesan cheese

salt and pepper to taste

1 cup fresh basil leaves

1 tbsp red wine vinegar

Directions:

Begin by heating a frying pan over a medium to high flame. After heating the pan put the almonds into the pan and let them cook for 4 to 5 minutes.

Once the almonds have reached a golden-brown color, place it into a food processor until you reach the consistency of fine powder.

Mix into the food processor the basil, red wine vinegar, and the tomatoes. Wait until the mixture becomes smooth and add the olive oil.

Continue processing for 35 seconds before adding the salt, pepper, and Parmesan. After a few pulses, the mix is ready to serve.

You can refrigerate for a cooler mix.

Nutrition:

Calories: 167

Carbohydrates: 18 g

Fats: 6 g

Proteins: 3 g

Marinated Olives with Feta

Difficulty Level: 2/5

Preparation time: 10 minutes

Cooking time: None

Servings: 4

Ingredients:

½ cup crumbled feta cheese

black pepper to taste

1 tsp grated lemon zest

2 cups pitted kalamata olives, drained and sliced

2 tbsp extra-virgin olive oil

2 tbsp lemon juice

2 garlic cloves, minced

Directions:

In a container, put together the feta cheese and olives. Toss the ingredients together along with olive oil.

After tossing mix together the garlic, lemon juice, and lemon zest. Add pepper and refrigerate before serving.

Nutrition:

Calories: 272

Carbohydrates: 48 g

Fats: 8 g

Proteins: 6 g

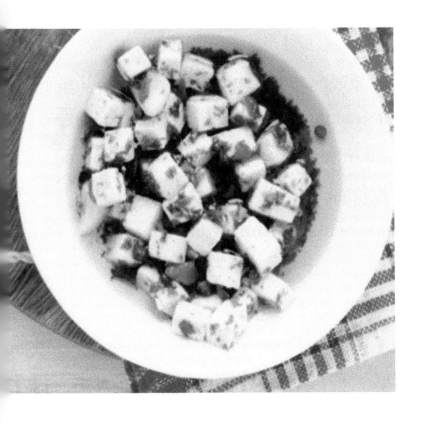

Healthy Nachos

Difficulty Level: 2/5

Preparation time: 10 minutes

Cooking time: 2 minutes

Servings: 6

Ingredients:

1 (4-oz) package finely crumbled feta cheese

1 finely chopped and drained plum tomato

1 medium green onion, thinly sliced (about 1 tbsp.)

2 tsp. oil from the container of sun-dried tomatoes

2 tbsp. sun-dried tomatoes in oil, finely chopped

2 tbsp. Kalamata olives, finely chopped

4 oz. restaurant-style corn tortilla chips

Directions:

Combine the plum tomato, sun-dried tomatoes, onion, olives, and oil into a container.

Microwave the tortilla chips along with the cheese for a minute on high settings. Rotate the plate 180 degrees before continuing to microwave for an additional 30 seconds.

After removing from the microwave, add the tomato mix and serve.

Nutrition:

Calories: 107

Carbohydrates: 20 g

Fats: 4 g

Proteins: 9 g

Stuffed Celery Bites

Difficulty Level: 2/5

Preparation time: 15 minutes

Cooking time: 4 minutes

Servings: 8

Ingredients:

Olive oil cooking spray

Celery leaves

¼ cup Italian cheese blend, shredded

1 (8-ounce) fat-free cream cheese

1 clove garlic, minced

2 tbsp. Pine nuts

2 tbsp. Sunflower seeds, dry-roasted

8 stalks celery

Procedure:

Prepare a frying pan by lightly coating it with olive oil. Over medium flame setting, add the pine nuts, garlic, and sauté for 4 minutes or until the pine nuts reach a golden-brown color.

Prepare the celery by removing the wide base and the tops. Then remove two strips from the side so as to make a flat surface.

In a container, mix together the cream cheese and Italian cheese. Spread the mixture on to the celery.

Cut the stalk into two-inch parts. Add pine nuts to half the cuts and sunflower seeds into the other half.

Cover the container and let it sit for 4 hours before serving.

Nutrition:

Calories: 57

Carbohydrates: 12 g

Fats: 2 g

Proteins: 5 g

Squash Fries

Difficulty Level: 2/5

Preparation time: 15 minutes

Cooking time: 10 minutes

Servings: 6

Ingredients:

½ tbsp. Grapeseed oil?

⅛ tsp. sea salt

1 medium butternut squash

1 tbsp. extra virgin olive oil

Directions:

Prepare the squash by peeling it. Remove the seeds before cutting into thin strips.

Place the strips into a container. Drizzle with grapeseed oil. Add virgin olive oil along with a pinch or two of salt.

Toss together the mix. Broil the mix in the oven until the squash turns crispy.

Nutrition:

Calories: 70

Carbohydrates: 27 g

Fats: 6 g

Proteins: 8 g

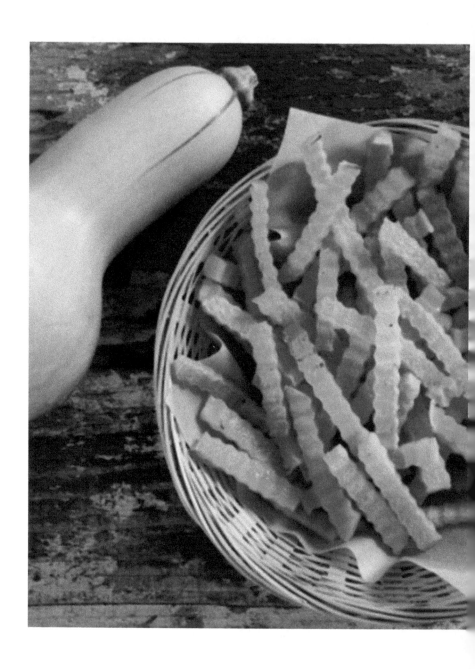

Avocado Toast

Difficulty Level: 2/5

Preparation time: 3

Cooking time: 7

Servings: 4

Ingredients:

A squeeze of fresh lemon juice, to taste

Sea salt and black pepper, to taste

2 ripe avocados, peeled

2 tbsp. freshly chopped mint, plus extra to garnish

4 large slices rye bread

80 grams soft feta, crumbled

Directions:

Mash the avocado using a fork and then add mint and lemon juice and continue mashing the avocado.

After being fully mashed, add the salt and black pepper to taste.

Prepare the bread by toasting or grilling it. Spread one-fourth of the avocado mix on each slice and add the Feta cheese at the top. Add mint before serving.

Nutrition:

Calories: 483

Carbohydrates 33 g

Fats: 68 g

Proteins: 12 g

Green Omelet

Difficulty Level: 2/5

Preparation time: 5 minutes

Cooking time: 10 minutes

Servings: 4

Ingredients:

½ cup Parmigiano-Reggiano cheese, grated

1 yellow onion, finely chopped

1 clove garlic, minced

1 medium bunch of collard greens

1 tsp. allspice

1 pinch sea salt, optional

3 tbsp. parsley, chopped

5 tbsp. extra virgin olive oil

8 eggs

Directions:

Start with beating the eggs and adding in the collard greens, parsley, garlic, onion, and allspice. Continue beating until all ingredients are mixed well.

Prepare a frying pan and place it over medium heat on the stove. Pour in the olive oil.

Add the mixture into the frying pan and continue cooking for 6 minutes on each side.

Serve while hot and sprinkle cheese for best results.

Nutrition:

Calories: 589

Carbohydrates: 30 g

Fats: 56 g

Proteins: 23 g

Mango Mug Cake

Difficulty Level: 2/5

Preparation time: 5 minutes

Cooking time: 10 minutes

Servings: 2

Ingredients

1 medium-sized mango, peeled and diced

2 eggs

1 teaspoon vanilla

1/4 teaspoon grated nutmeg

1 tablespoon cocoa powder

2 tablespoons honey

1/2 cup coconut flour

Directions:

Combine the coconut flour, eggs, honey, vanilla, nutmeg and cocoa powder in two lightly greased mugs.

Then, add 1 cup of water and a metal trivet to the Pressure pot. Lower the uncovered mugs onto the trivet.

Secure the lid. Choose the "Manual" mode and High pressure; cook for 10 minutes. Once cooking is complete, use a quick pressure release; carefully remove the lid.

Top with diced mango and serve chilled. Enjoy!

Nutrition:

Calories 268;

Fat 10.5g;

Carbohydrates 34.8g;

Protein 10.6g;

Sugars 31.1g

Chocolate Coffee Pots de Crème

Difficulty Level: 2/5

Preparation time: 10 minutes

Cooking time: 15 minutes

Servings: 6

Ingredients:

1 teaspoon instant coffee

9 ounces chocolate chips

1/2 cup whole milk

1/3 cup sugar

A pinch of pink salt

4 egg yolks

2 cups double cream

Directions:

Place a metal trivet and 1 cup of water in your Pressure pot.

In a saucepan, bring the cream and milk to a simmer.

Then, thoroughly combine the egg yolks, sugar, instant coffee, and salt. Slowly and gradually whisk in the hot cream mixture.

Whisk in the chocolate chips and blend again. Pour the mixture into mason jars. Lower the jars onto the trivet.

Secure the lid. Choose the "Manual" mode and cook for 6 minutes at High pressure. Once cooking is complete, use a natural pressure release for 10 minutes; carefully remove the lid.

Serve well chilled and enjoy!

Nutrition:

Calories 351;

Fat 19.3g;

Carbohydrates 39.3g;

Protein 5.5g;

Sugars 32.1g

Almond Cherry Crumble Cake

Difficulty Level: 2/5

Preparation time: 5 minutes
Cooking time: 10 minutes
Servings: 4

Ingredients

1/4 cup almonds, slivered

1/2 stick butter, at room temperature

1 teaspoon ground cinnamon

A pinch of grated nutmeg

1 cup rolled oats

1/3 teaspoon ground cardamom

1 teaspoon pure vanilla extract

1/3 cup honey

2 tablespoons all-purpose flour

A pinch of salt

1-pound sweet cherries, pitted

1/3 cup water

Directions

Arrange the cherries on the bottom of the Pressure pot. Sprinkle cinnamon, cardamom, and vanilla over the top. Add the water and honey.

In a separate mixing bowl, thoroughly combine the butter, oats, and flour. Spread topping mixture evenly over cherry mixture.

Secure the lid. Choose the "Manual" mode and High pressure; cook for 10 minutes. Once cooking is complete, use a natural pressure release; carefully remove the lid.

Serve at room temperature. Bon appétit!

Nutrition:

Calories 335;

Fat 13.4g;

Carbohydrates 60.5g;

Protein 5.9g;

Sugars 38.1g

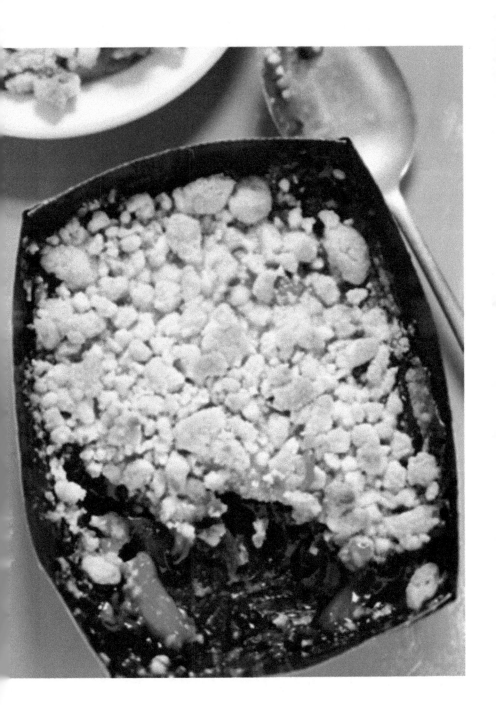

Orange Butterscotch Pudding

Difficulty Level: 2/5

Preparation time: 10 minutes

Cooking time: 15 minutes

Servings: 4

Ingredients:

4 caramels

2 eggs, well-beaten

1/4 cup freshly squeezed orange juice

1/3 cup sugar

1 cup cake flour

1/2 teaspoon baking powder

1/4 cup milk

1 stick butter, melted

1/2 teaspoon vanilla essence

Sauce:

1/2 cup golden syrup

2 teaspoons corn flour

1 cup boiling water

Directions:

Melt the butter and milk in the microwave. Whisk in the eggs, vanilla, and sugar. After that, stir in the flour, baking powder, and orange juice.

Lastly, add the caramels and stir until everything is well combined and melted.

Divide between the four jars. Add 1 ½ cups of water and a metal trivet to the bottom of the Pressure pot. Lower the jars onto the trivet.

To make the sauce, whisk the boiling water, corn flour, and golden syrup until everything is well combined. Pour the sauce into each jar.

Secure the lid. Choose the "Steam" mode and cook for 15 minutes under High pressure. Once cooking is complete, use a natural pressure release; carefully remove the lid. Enjoy!

Nutrition:

Calories 565;

Fat 25.9g;

Carbohydrates 79.6g;

Protein 6.4g;

Sugars 51.5g

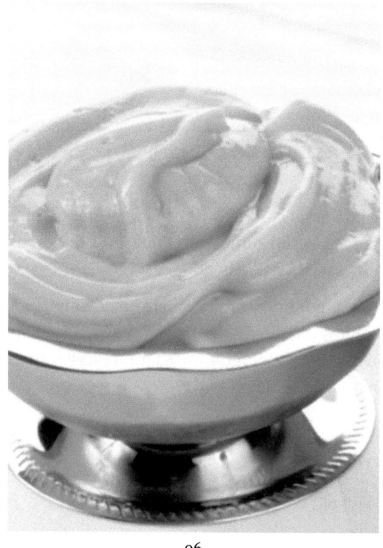

Recipe for Ruby Pears Delight

Difficulty Level: 2/5

Preparation time: 10 minutes

Cooking time: 10 minutes

Servings: 4

Ingredients:

4 Pears

Grape juice-26 oz.

Currant jelly-11 oz.

4 garlic cloves

Juice and zest of 1 lemon

4 peppercorns

2 rosemary springs

1/2 vanilla bean

Directions:

Pour the jelly and grape juice in your pressure pot and mix with lemon zest and juice

In the mix, dip each pear and wrap them in a clean tin foil and place them orderly in the steamer basket of your pressure pot

Combine peppercorns, rosemary, garlic cloves and vanilla bean to the juice mixture,

Seal the lid and cook at High for 10 minutes.

Release the pressure quickly, and carefully open the lid; bring out the pears, remove wrappers and arrange them on plates. Serve when cold with toppings of cooking juice.

Nutrition:

Calories: 145

Fat: 5.6

Fiber: 6

Carbs: 12

Protein: 12

Mixed Berry and Orange Compote

Difficulty Level: 2/5

Preparation time: 15 minutes

Cooking time: 15 minutes

Servings: 4

Ingredients:

1/2-pound strawberries

1 tablespoon orange juice

1/4 teaspoon ground cloves

1/2 cup brown sugar

1 vanilla bean

1-pound blueberries

1/2-pound blackberries

Directions:

Place your berries in the inner pot. Add the sugar and let sit for 15 minutes. Add in the orange juice, ground cloves, and vanilla bean.

Secure the lid. Choose the "Manual" mode and cook for 2 minutes at High pressure. Once cooking is complete, use a natural pressure release for 10 minutes; carefully remove the lid.

As your compote cools, it will thicken. Bon appétit!

Nutrition:

Calories 224;

Fat 0.8g;

Carbohydrates 56.3g;

Protein 2.1g;

Sugars 46.5g

Streuselkuchen with Peaches

Difficulty Level: 2/5

Preparation time: 10 minutes

Cooking time: 20 minutes

Servings: 6

Ingredients

1 cup rolled oats

1 teaspoon vanilla extract

1/3 cup orange juice

4 tablespoons raisins

2 tablespoons honey

4 tablespoons butter

4 tablespoons all-purpose flour

A pinch of grated nutmeg

1/2 teaspoon ground cardamom

A pinch of salt

1 teaspoon ground cinnamon

6 peaches, pitted and chopped

1/3 cup brown sugar

Directions:

Place the peaches on the bottom of the inner pot. Sprinkle with the cardamom, cinnamon and vanilla. Top with the orange juice, honey, and raisins.

In a mixing bowl, whisk together the butter, oats, flour, brown sugar, nutmeg, and salt. Drop by a spoonful on top of the peaches.

Secure the lid. Choose the "Manual" mode and cook for 8 minutes at High pressure. Once cooking is complete, use a natural pressure release for 10 minutes; carefully remove the lid. Bon appétit!

Nutrition:

329 Calories;

10g Fat;

56g Carbohydrates;

6.9g Protein;

31g Sugars

Fig and Homey Buckwheat Pudding

Difficulty Level: 2/5

Preparation time: 10 minutes

Cooking time: 10 minutes

Servings: 4

Ingredients

1/2 teaspoon ground cinnamon

1/2 cup dried figs, chopped

1/3 cup honey

1 teaspoon pure vanilla extract

3 ½ cups milk

1/2 teaspoon pure almond extract

1 ½ cups buckwheat

Directions:

Add all of the above ingredients to your Pressure pot.

Secure the lid. Choose the "Multigrain" mode and cook for 10 minutes under High pressure. Once cooking is complete, use a natural pressure release; carefully remove the lid.

Serve topped with fresh fruits, nuts or whipped topping. Bon appétit!

Nutrition:

Calories 320;

Fat 7.5g;

Carbohydrates 57.7g;

Protein 9.5g;

Sugars 43.2g

Zingy Blueberry Sauce

Difficulty Level: 2/5

Preparation time: 5 minutes

Cooking time: 20 minutes

Servings: 10

Ingredients

1/4 cup fresh lemon juice

1-pound granulated sugar

1 tablespoon freshly grated lemon zest

1/2 teaspoon vanilla extract

2 pounds fresh blueberries

Directions:

Place the blueberries, sugar, and vanilla in the inner pot of your Pressure pot.

Secure the lid. Choose the "Manual" mode and cook for 2 minutes at High pressure. Once cooking is complete, use a natural pressure release for 15 minutes; carefully remove the lid.

Stir in the lemon zest and juice. Puree in a food processor; then, strain and push the mixture through a sieve before storing. Enjoy!

Nutrition:

Calories 230;

Fat 0.3g;

Carbohydrates 59g;

Protein 0.7g;

Sugars 53.6g

Chocolate Almond Custard

Difficulty Level: 2/5

Preparation time: 10 minutes

Cooking time: 15 minutes

Servings: 3

Ingredients

3 chocolate cookies, chunks

A pinch of salt

1/4 teaspoon ground cardamom

3 tablespoons honey

1/4 teaspoon freshly grated nutmeg

2 tablespoons butter

3 tablespoons whole milk

1 cup almond flour

3 eggs

1 teaspoon pure vanilla extract

Directions:

In a mixing bowl, beat the eggs with butter. Now, add the milk and continue mixing until well combined.

Add the remaining ingredients in the order listed above. Divide the batter among 3 ramekins.

Add 1 cup of water and a metal trivet to the Pressure pot. Cover ramekins with foil and lower them onto the trivet.

Secure the lid and select "Manual" mode. Cook at High pressure for 12 minutes. Once cooking is complete, use a quick release; carefully remove the lid.

Transfer the ramekins to a wire rack and allow them to cool slightly before serving. Enjoy!

Nutrition:

Calories 304;

Fat 18.9g;

Carbohydrates 23.8g;

Protein 10g;

Sugars 21.1g

Honey Stewed Apples

Difficulty Level: 2/5

Preparation time: 5 minutes

Cooking time: 5 minutes

Servings: 4

Ingredients

2 tablespoons honey

1 teaspoon ground cinnamon

1/2 teaspoon ground cloves

4 apples

Directions

Add all ingredients to the inner pot. Now, pour in 1/3 cup of water.

Secure the lid. Choose the "Manual" mode and cook for 2 minutes at High pressure. Once cooking is complete, use a quick pressure release; carefully remove the lid.

Serve in individual bowls. Bon appétit!

Nutrition:

Calories 128;

Fat 0.3g;

Carbohydrates 34.3g;

Protein 0.5g;

Sugars 27.5g

Greek-Style Compote with Yogurt

Difficulty Level: 2/5

Preparation time: 5 minutes

Cooking time: 15 minutes

Servings: 4

Ingredients:

1 cup Greek yoghurt

1 cup pears

4 tablespoons honey

1 cup apples

1 vanilla bean

1 cinnamon stick

1/2 cup caster sugar

1 cup rhubarb

1 teaspoon ground ginger

1 cup plums

Directions:

Place the fruits, ginger, vanilla, cinnamon, and caster sugar in the inner pot of your Pressure pot.

Secure the lid. Choose the "Manual" mode and cook for 2 minutes at High pressure. Once cooking is complete, use a natural pressure release for 10 minutes; carefully remove the lid.

Meanwhile, whisk the yogurt with the honey.

Serve your compote in individual bowls with a dollop of honeyed Greek yogurt. Enjoy!

Nutrition:

Calories 304;

Fat 0.3g;

Carbohydrates 75.4g;

Protein 5.1g;

Sugars 69.2g

Lightning Source UK Ltd.
Milton Keynes UK
UKHW020703310521
384670UK00006B/132

9 781802 7745